Chair Exercises for Fall Prevention

Also by Amanda Sterczyk

Pace Yourself: Exercising After COVID-19

Sweat-Free Exercises for the Office

Balance Exercises for Fall Prevention

Balance 2.0: Preventing Falls with Exercise

Your Job Is Killing You:
A User's Guide to Sneaking Exercise into Your Work Day

Balance and Your Body:
How Exercise Can Help You Avoid a Fall

Move More, Your Life Depends On It:
Practical Tips to Add More Movement to Your Day

I Can See Your Underwear:
My Journey Through the Fitness World

Fiction:

Selfried and the Secrets: A Novel

For more information,
please visit amandasterczyk.com.

Chair Exercises for Fall Prevention

Amanda Sterczyk, MA, CPT

The information in this book should not be used for diagnosis or treatment, or as a substitute for professional medical care. Before beginning any exercise program, consult your physician.

Copyright © Amanda Sterczyk 2022

All rights reserved. No part of this publication may be reproduced, stored in a retrieval system or transmitted in any form or by any means without the prior written permission of the author, nor be otherwise circulated in any form of binding or cover other than that in which it is published and without a similar condition being imposed on the purchaser.

   Excerpt from "How I felt after 70 days of lying in bed for science," *Vice Magazine* © 2015 Andrew Iwanicki. Reproduced with permission. All rights reserved.
   Excerpt from "Rating of Perceived Exertion Scale," published by Productive Fitness © 2017. Used with permission. All rights reserved.

Sterczyk, Amanda, author
   Chair Exercises for Fall Prevention.

Includes bibliographical references.
Issued in print and electronic formats.

ISBN 9798772565926

   1. Aging. 2. Fall Prevention 3. Physical Fitness 4. Healthy Aging 5. Balance Training

Editor: Kaarina Stiff
Cover image: iStock Photo
Image credit: ankomando
Exercise illustrations: Emily Sterczyk
Layout: Matthew Bin
Published by Kindle Direct Publishing

May you live a long and healthy life,

free from slips, trips, and broken hips.

And falls.

Move more, feel better.

CONTENTS

Introduction	1
Chapter One: Falling and the Basics of Balance	5
Is Fear a Vicious Circle?	7
Have You Ever Fallen?	7
What's the Problem with Falling?	9
How's Your Balance?	11
Do You Know about the Heel-Toe Express?	13
What's Gravity Got to Do With It?	14
Do You Know the Three Pillars of Balance?	17
How Does Your Posture Impact Your Fall Risk?	18
Do You Play the Piano?	19
Sarco-what?	21
Are You a Well-Oiled Machine?	22
Do You Play with CARs?	23
Chapter Two: Exercise Setup	25
May I Remain Seated?	27
The Safety Talk	27
Setting Up Your Space to Exercise	28
Exercising at the Right Level	29
How to Approach the Exercises	31
Balance Definitions	33
What's the Speed Limit?	34
Please Keep Breathing	35
Don't Forget to Warmup	35
Chapter Three: The Exercises	37
Rating of Perceived Exertion (RPE) Scale	39
Active Sitting	40

Seated Finger Follow	42
Seated Joint Mobility	44
Neck	45
Shoulders	46
Elbows	47
Wrists	48
Fingers	49
Waist	51
Ankles	52
Seated Clock Toe Taps	54
Double Gas Pedal	56
Heel Slides	58
Torso Twists	60
Reverse Sit-ups	62
Side to Side Arm Reaches	64
Seated Overhead Arm Raises	66
Seated Wall Push-up	68
Seated Side Bends	70
Seated Knee Straightener	72
Seated High March	74
Appendix: Exercise Breakdown, Sample Workouts, & Activity Logs	77
Checking In With Yourself	81
Reviews and Testimonials	89
About the Author	91

Introduction

As we age, we tend to slow down. Our muscles shrink, our vision blurs, and our reaction time diminishes. Together, all of these factors lead to an increased risk of falling. But it doesn't need to be that way. This book provides an exercise guide to keep your muscles strong and your confidence high. We all need bodies that will support our weight as we move through life. Our confidence in our ability to maintain an upright position—i.e., to *not* fall—is just as important.

My hope with my balance books is to rebuild your confidence *and* your muscles, so that you can enjoy your golden years. You deserve as much, and I want to help you get there.

This book is different than my other *Balance* exercise guides, in that all of the exercises are completed while seated. They still address your balance system, strength, posture, and joint mobility. But you can (and should) remain seated when you follow along to complete your balance workout. The exercises will still improve walking, reinforce good posture, and enhance ease of movement during your day-to-day life.

This book is an exercise guide. I'm sharing with you fundamental exercises that will help you increase strength and flexibility, at the same time that you're working on posture and balance. I've also created a series of workout plans, to help guide you through four workouts. But you can also dive in and tackle the exercises in the order in which they appear. It's up to you, either option will provide benefits.

What hasn't changed in this book is the degree of explanation for each exercise. It begins with a summary table of exercise by fall prevention goal—be it balance, posture, strength, and/or flexibility (these mini tables are also summarized together at the end of the book). You will receive set up instructions on how to start, step-by-step instructions, and recommendations to make each exercise easier or harder (while still remaining seated, of course). Most of the exercises also include guidance on how to visualize the movement, to further build linkages between your brain and body.

You will notice that the exercises only feature very basic illustrations to guide you. That's on purpose, and it's the same reason why not every exercise features a visualization cue. Often, people rush through movements (aka exercise sequences) if they *think* they know what's next, or if they don't like a particular move. I've seen it dozens (even hundreds) of times when I've been teaching group fitness classes or training individuals in their homes. I'm here to say, please don't rush the movement. Use your time with this book to focus on your body, be mindful of how you're moving, and use muscle power—not momentum—to complete the sequences. In an effort to slow you down, I'm asking you to do more work to understand and execute the movements. This added work has an added bonus—it's helping keep your brain healthy too.

I hope you enjoy this book.

Chapter One:
Falling and the Basics of Balance

Amanda Sterczyk

Is Fear a Vicious Circle?

Fear of falling keeps some people from getting up and moving more. Does this feel familiar? Unfortunately, lack of movement further weakens our muscles, stiffens our joints, and reduces our ability to balance. I've seen it many times: A senior has a fall and injures themselves. As they recover from their injury, they become less mobile and sure-footed, so they move less. Then the movement feels forced and unnatural, which further saps their confidence, so they move even less. Then their bodies become weaker, stiffer, and more unbalanced, so they move less still.

Can you relate to this scenario? A single fall can undermine your confidence and impact your activity level. Thus begins the vicious cycle of falls. With this book, I want to build your confidence. I want to show you that there are safe ways to strengthen your body and improve your balance, even whilst sitting down. It's what I do with my senior clients during fitness house calls.

Have You Ever Fallen?

Have you ever fallen? I have fallen more than once, but one fall in particular stands out in my head. It was a dark winter evening, and the walking conditions were less than ideal. I was heading out back to our car. Just as I passed the garage, I slipped on the ice and fell. Try as I might, I couldn't stand up on the slippery driveway.

Even though I was only about 30 feet from our back door, I knew I needed help. I pulled out my cell phone and called our home phone.

"I've fallen and I can't get up." Sound familiar? It reminded me of a television commercial I first saw as a child. You might remember it too. In it, an older, grey-haired woman uttered the phrase from her bathroom floor. While I may have had some grey hairs peeking around the edges, I was only 43 years old when I said it.

As I waited for my kids to come to my rescue — they arrived quite quickly, actually, but still lovingly tease me about it to this day — I thought of how many seniors fall at home, just like in the commercial. And they don't always have someone who can help them.

As a fitness professional, I realized that I could help seniors take charge of their lives and reduce their risk of falling. While you'll need to consult with Mother Nature and municipal road crews about the state of icy sidewalks in the winter, I can help you improve your balance, strength, and mobility to decrease the likelihood of falling both in your home and when you're out and about — ice and snow being the exception, of course. Exercise works wonders to help you avoid a fall.

What's the Problem with Falling?

As we age, our risk of falling increases, as does the likelihood that a fall will cause an injury. In Canada, falls are the leading cause of injury among older Canadians. Twenty to thirty percent of seniors experience one or more falls each year. Falls are the cause of 85 percent of seniors' injury-related hospitalizations. You may be surprised to learn that falls are the cause of 95 percent of all hip fractures and fully half of all falls causing hospitalization happen at home.[1]

In the United States, data reported by the National Council on Aging show that one quarter of Americans over the age of 65 will fall each year. Falls are also the prevailing reason for hospital admissions among the elderly. An emergency room in the United States treats a senior fall victim every 11 seconds. And if you're an older adult, you're more likely to die from a fall than any other cause.[2]

---

[1] Public Health Agency of Canada, You CAN Prevent Falls! (Ottawa: Government of Canada, 2005, Revised 2015), https://www.canada.ca/en/public-health/services/health-promotion/aging-seniors/publications/publications-general-public/you-prevent-falls.html. Reprinted with permission from the Minister of Health, 2019.

[2] National Council on Aging (website), Falls Prevention Facts, accessed March 22, 2019, https://www.ncoa.org/news/resources-for-reporters/get-the-facts/falls-prevention-facts/.

In the past, research attributed the risk of falls exclusively to aging. That is to say, the likelihood of a fall was simply connected to the year we were born. In fact, it's more like aging and lack of physical activity are working together to increase the likelihood that we will fall. As we age, we are typically less active. Our bodies get weaker, our bones get more brittle, and that is why we're more likely to fall. And when we do suffer a fall later in life, we're also more likely to be injured.

Researcher and professor Robert Wood is featured in a YouTube video called "Why Seniors Fall."[3] In the video, Wood offers simple tips for exercises that can be incorporated into your daily routine, such as drawing the letters of the alphabet with your foot. This helps increase flexibility in your ankle and strengthen the muscles up your shin, which are both important to help you lift your foot as you walk, and thus prevent a fall. My mother was the one who first alerted me to Dr. Wood's terrific video because, as she said, "It's just like all the exercises you have us do in your exercise class."

She was right. Dr. Wood's video demonstrated fundamental exercises that equip seniors with muscular strength and good balance. I focus on similar skills

---

[3] Robert Wood, "Why Seniors Fall," *Electronic Caregiver* (March 29, 2012), https://www.youtube.com/watch?v=T5x6kTrwgYw.

in my exercise classes and one-on-one sessions with seniors.

How's Your Balance?

Think about your current health. How's your balance? Can you close your eyes whilst standing on one leg? If so, can you hold that pose for 15 to 30 seconds? Most adults don't even realize their balance has deteriorated until after they fall and hurt themselves. And let me tell you, falling is not age-specific. However, as we age, our chances of experiencing a fall increase drastically. And as we discussed earlier, you're more likely to be injured from a fall the older you are.

We all need good balance to safely move around our world on a daily basis, but it's easy to take it for granted. If you've ever lost your balance, fallen, and sustained an injury, you get it. Balance is a critical component of walking, which is basically just a process of transferring our weight from side to side and maintaining an upright posture. With each step, we shift our weight from one foot to the other. If you have trouble with balance, then it makes sense that you would also have trouble walking. And it's when you're walking that you're most likely to fall.

If balance is a challenge for you, you're likely more aware of the importance of being able to maintain an upright position without falling over. It's cute when a toddler is learning to walk and they tip over. A young child falls regularly, but over time, their balance improves and they fall less often. As adults age, poor balance can be life-threatening and, quite frankly, frightening.

Whether we like it or not, as we get older, our balance is negatively impacted by our aging bodies. Let's take a closer look at what our bodies are going through:

- Cells die in our vestibular system, which is connected to the part of our brain that controls balance.
- Our vision declines and with it, our depth perception.
- Changes to our blood pressure may cause dizziness, light-headedness or blurriness.
- We lose muscle mass, strength, and power, which can slow our reaction time if we trip.
- Our reflexes and coordination decline.
- A variety of health problems can impact our balance, including arthritis, stroke, Parkinson's disease and multiple sclerosis.[4]

---

[4] Anthony Komaroff, "Why does balance decline with age?" Ask Dr. K/Harvard Health Publications (website), accessed September 22, 2018, https://www.askdoctork.com/why-does-balance-decline-with-age-201306054928.

Regular physical activity is the key to maintaining good balance. An exercise program that focuses on specific balance exercises as well as core strengthening and movement patterns will improve balance and stability, not to mention daily function. The exercises in this book are geared to helping you avoid a fall. I hope you'll see that exercise does not need to be complicated.

Do You Know about the Heel-Toe Express?

Walking is the main form of physical activity for many older adults. It's a great low-cost, uncomplicated way to stay active. And proper walking form can achieve all of the fitness goals that will help prevent a slip, trip, or fall.

As we discussed in the last section, walking is essentially a dynamic balance exercise: you constantly shift your weight from one foot to the other and back again. To successfully accomplish this dynamic balance work, your muscles need to be strong enough to continuously lift your feet and clear the ground safely. Your bones and muscles in your torso must be strong enough to maintain an upright posture. And your balance is being continuously challenged as you shift your centre of gravity and base of support (more on those concepts later).

Ironically, though, walking is when most falls occur because one or more of these components is coming up short. But there's an easy fix, and if you keep reading I'll show you.

What's Gravity Got to Do With It?

What do astronauts on the International Space Station have in common with someone who is bed-ridden with an illness or injury? It's not a trick question. The answer is "no gravity." Being horizontal for extended periods of time impacts bodily functions, so much so that NASA paid test subjects $18,000 to lie in bed for 70 days while being poked, prodded, and monitored.[5] Then they asked them to try standing up for 15 minutes. It sounds easy enough, but it wasn't.

Our bodies don't like to be sedentary for very long. After a while, our organs and systems start to decay. This can include decreased blood volume, reduced bone density, loss of muscle strength, disappearance of fine and gross motor skills, and vanishing balance and mobility. Our hearts have to pump harder to move blood throughout our bodies, bed

---

[5] Andrew Iwanicki, "How I felt after 70 days of lying in bed for science," *Vice Magazine*, Feb. 5, 2015, https://www.vice.com/en_us/article/jma83d/nasa-patient-8179-200.

sores can develop on our skin, and our emotional well-being also takes a hit.[6]

The NASA study was an effort to assess the physiological impact of extended space travel to Mars, but, as with many NASA initiatives, the results have real-world implications on Earth right now. How can older adults with physical limitations and mobility issues maintain independence while fighting the effects of zero-gravity from extended sedentary time?

Mobility is critical for maintaining independence and for keeping costly, long-term care services to a minimum. According to researchers in the United States, a six-month delay in entering a nursing home can reduce health care costs by millions.[7] These same researchers are working to identify older adults who are at risk of disability and creating customized exercise programs to prevent an inevitable downward slide. And guess what they're focusing on in terms of activity? The strength and balance required to lift one

---

[6] Kimberly Turtenwald, "The effects of immobility on the body systems," AZCentral (website) accessed Feb 7, 2015, https://healthyliving.azcentral.com/the-effects-of-immobility-on-the-body-systems-12497238.html.

[7] Kay Lazar, "Fitness for elders is key, study finds," *Boston Globe*, January 24, 2015, https://www.bostonglobe.com/metro/2015/01/24/researchers-redouble-efforts-understand-and-improve-elders-mobility-problems/HoU5skivE2wvsGvT1H38ZO/story.html

foot after the other, whether it's to climb the stairs or to simply walk *to* those stairs.

Here's how one of the NASA research participants described his first walk after 70 days in bed: "With a staff member on each side…I sat up on the stretcher and stepped down onto the ground. My feet tingled like they were sluggish and short as I dragged my feet across the ground and kicked my ankles. I lacked all the fine coordination skills that I hadn't used for months. I felt sharp pains in my ankles and feet as I pivoted through the obstacle course, and I certainly couldn't walk a straight line well." It didn't last, though: "Within a few days of casual strolling and formal reconditioning exercise, my balance returned and my endurance began to recover."[8]

Bottom line, if you experience an extended period of time in a horizontal position — bed-ridden — please make an effort to get out of bed and let gravity work on your body. You can do this by sitting on your bed and begin moving your arms and legs. Next, try standing next to your bed. Then, you can slowly increase movement and activity every day. It's not too late, and your body will thank you for it. Every movement you make will work towards improving your

---

[8] Andrew Iwanicki, "How I felt after 70 days of lying in bed for science." Reprinted with permission.

balance. And strengthening your balance system is key to preventing falls, so we'll cover that next.

Do You Know the Three Pillars of Balance?

Our balance system is complex and relies on sensory input from three distinct systems: visual, vestibular, and proprioceptive (also known as somatosensory). All of this is just a fancy way of describing how our bodies process information.[9] Let me break them down.

Visual system: As you might guess, this is about our eyes, which provide visual input to our brains as we move through life.

Vestibular system: This is the medical term for the inner ear, which processes sensory information about motion, equilibrium, and spatial orientation. Close your eyes and slowly move your head side to side. Your vestibular system is now sending crucial input to your brain. As we age, our side-to-side head movements become less frequent, which negatively impacts our vestibular system. In other words, it doesn't work if we don't use it. "Use it or lose it" doesn't just apply to our muscles — it applies to every single part of our bodies.

---

[9] Physiopedia (website), Balance, accessed March 27, 2019, https://www.physiopedia.com/Balance.

Proprioception or somatosensory: This is our brain's ability to sense our body's position in space. That's why we can walk through our house in the dark without falling down, unless of course, we bang into an unseen object. The nerves in our body send signals to our brain that allow us to maintain an upright position, and we have just as many sensors (i.e., nerve endings) in the bottom of our feet as we do in our entire spinal column. The nerve endings in our spinal column rely on posture to determine our body's orientation as it moves. That's why posture is a key component of balance and preventing falls, and why working on your posture whilst seated is just as important as your standing posture.

How Does Your Posture Impact Your Fall Risk?

When you have a stooped posture — whether it's due to weak muscles, too much sitting, or years of slouching forward at a desk — your centre of gravity is no longer over your base of support. In this case, if you catch your foot on something and slip, momentum will propel you forward. And it's very difficult to pull yourself back and up once momentum takes over.

In this hunched-over position, your bones are not aligned, and you can't support your body weight. Instead, your muscles and your connective tissue — the tendons that connect muscles to bones and ligaments that connect bones to each other — have been assigned a role that's normally reserved for your bones. Eventually, these muscles, tendons, and ligaments declare a strike because they already have a job to do. They don't want a second job. It's like asking the widget makers to also make sprockets; they'd rather stick to making widgets and let the sprocket makers make the sprockets.

Think of your body as a finely-tuned, highly specialized assembly line. Every part of our body is designed for its specialty. If you don't use all the parts in the right way, they'll stop functioning. In the case of movement, if you're going to keep moving, other parts will have to jump in and help. And that's when you risk falling.

It's not too late to start. Your body has an incredible feedback loop of action-reaction. If you begin to work your muscles and load your bones, your body will respond. But if you don't use them, you will lose them.

Do You Play the Piano?

A *long* time ago, when I was in the seventh grade, my teacher commented on how good a fellow student's posture was. Even though most of us were bored with the lesson, this student was sitting completely upright. The rest of us were either slumped over our desks with our eyes just inches from our worksheet or leaning against the chair's backrest.

The teacher continued to praise her and exclaimed, "You must take piano lessons! I can tell someone has drilled into you the importance of good posture." I guiltily sat upright at that point; my organ teacher was regularly chastising me for slouching during our lessons.

Your piano (or organ) teacher was right. Or maybe it was your mother who told you to sit up straight. If you are holding your body upright instead of relying on furniture, your muscles are working. Many of us outsource the job of our muscles to our chairs when we constantly slouch instead of sitting more actively.

How do you sit in a chair? Do you make your muscles hold you in an upright position, or have you outsourced their role to the furniture by slumping backwards?

To sit actively, we need to load our muscles and bones to fight the effects of gravity, and we must avoid outsourcing the role of our muscles by slumping in our seats. If you're hunched forward in your upper spine, your lower spine is probably tucked under, causing painful and unnecessary loading of the muscles, tendons, and ligaments.

Learning how to sit actively will engage muscles and load bones. It will improve posture, breathing, and mood, and it will make you stronger. Imagine that: sitting as a form of exercise. At the end of one fitness house call, my client Cynthia said to me, "It's amazing you can still work your body in a chair. I feel wonderful."

Sarco-what?

No one sets out to get weak. It just happens. And the problem is that our own bodies sometimes work against us. As we celebrate more birthdays, sarcopenia takes more of our strength. If you're thinking "sarco-what?!", let me elaborate.

Sarcopenia is age-related muscle loss that contributes to frailty, loss of strength, and inevitably, falls.[10] This decline begins in our 40s and follows a fairly straight pattern—each year, we lose more muscle. Have you noticed your legs getting skinnier, more spindly, every year? That's what sarcopenia looks like. By the time you're in your seventies, you've lost half the mass in your muscles.

One of the best ways to fight this loss of muscle tissue is with resistance or strength training.[11] Lower

---

[10]. Jeremy Walston, "Sarcopenia in Older Adults," *Curr Opin Rheumatol*, 26, no. 6 (November 2012): 623-627, 10.1097/BOR.0b013e328358d59b.

[11]. Walston, "Sarcopenia," 2012.

limb strength means your legs are able to carry you as you stand and walk. Those same legs need to be strong enough to step up to climb stairs, balance you as you shift weight from one foot to the other when you walk, and when you move from sitting to standing. Your upper body also needs to be strong in order to hold you upright and resist momentum and gravity, which would topple you over if you stoop too far forward. These upper body muscles also help you maintain an upright posture as you reach, twist, or turn during your everyday activities.

The targeted exercises included in this book will help you strengthen both your lower limbs and upper body muscles, which goes a long way to fighting back against sarcopenia.

Are You a Well-Oiled Machine?

When you move, do you feel as stiff as a robot? Does the feeling fade over time? If it fades, that's a good sign because the movement you're doing is helping to lubricate your joints. I'm here to tell you that you need to do more of it.

Joints are the connections between our bones, where two or more bones meet. Our muscles pull our bones towards or away from joints, depending on the movement we're doing. Spoiler alert: our muscles do all the work, and our bones and joints are just along for the ride. But when those joints aren't being used, such as when we're less active, the joints dry up.

If you're feeling particularly stiff and creaky one day and you have to speed up — for instance, if you're crossing the street and the light changes midway through your curb-to-curb excursion — stiff joints will make it difficult for you to act quickly. Your body may feel like a robot trying to ride a bicycle. Although the parts are moving, it looks forced and unnatural, and your reaction time is slower when those joints are rigid and dry. This rigidity and slower feedback between your body and your brain put you at greater risk of a fall.

But there's an easy fix. Has a health or fitness professional ever told you that motion is lotion? Or that movement is medicine? I'm guilty of using those phrases because they are effective ways to remind people that their bodies — including their joints — need and crave movement. And slow-motion, circular movements are the key to this lock.[12]

Do You Play with CARs?

My philosophy is the slower the movement, the better. Large rotations and circles performed s-l-o-w-l-y to follow all the possible angles at which each joint can move. And there's a great acronym to help you

---

[12] Meg Selig, "Is it true that 'Movement is medicine'?," *Psychology Today*, March 30, 2017, https://www.psychologytoday.com/us/blog/changepower/201703/is-it-true-movement-is-medicine.

remember what you need to do: CARs. I'll let certified athletic trainer Cassandra McCoy explain them: "CARs means Controlled Articular Rotations. As you do the exercise, you are making controlled movements within each joint articulation against gravity via a big rotation. The best thing is the more that you do them, the stronger you get, and the bigger your circle will become. You can start out with a baby circle working within your current range and then gradually, as you get stronger, that range of motion will get bigger."[13]

Having a limited range of motion in our joints can cause fear, because we're worried what will happen *if* we have to move quickly. So the key is to increase the range of our joints slowly, to allay our fears and increase our confidence. With CARs, we draw bigger and bigger circles in a controlled manner. Circles are 360 degrees; we have 360 joints in our body. And with all this talk of circles, it's time for me to tell you we've come full circle with our discussion of balance, strength, and mobility. Now it's time to move on to the action of improving balance.

---

[13] Excerpt from an interview with Cassandra McCoy, ATC, LAT, conducted via video chat and email on April 6, 2019.

Chapter Two: Exercise Setup

May I Remain Seated?

The exercises in this book have you seated for the duration of your workout. And that's on purpose. Chair exercises come in handy when you have limited mobility or find it hard to maintain your balance.

When you do chair exercises daily, you reduce the risk of falls. The movements increase blood flow and keep your joints active and lubricated. They also strengthen your muscles and increase your confidence when you do have to stand up and move around. Bottom line, you're improving your balance whilst seated. So don't feel shy about these chair exercises, take pride in the work you're doing to maintain your independence!

The Safety Talk

Before we proceed, let's talk about safety. As with other fitness texts, my book includes a disclaimer in the front: "The information in this book should not be used for diagnosis or treatment, or as a substitute for professional medical care. Before beginning any exercise program, consult your physician." That's not just legal jargon for the sake of it—it's important advice to heed because everyone's health is different.

But there's more: I want you to use your common sense. The exercises in this book are meant to help you, not hurt you. If something bothers you, STOP doing it.

If you have any questions at all about the exercises listed here, take this book to your doctor or other health professional and review it with them. Or you can hire a personal trainer in your neighbourhood to work with you. There are many great fitness professionals who work with older adults just like you.

And remember, the goal is to make you stronger and improve your balance. Even small increments of activity and exercise will get you closer to this goal.

Setting Up Your Space to Exercise

These are exercises you can do in your home—with your doctor's permission, of course. As you start each exercise, focus on making slow, purposeful movements. Even though you are sitting down for these exercises, you still need to gauge how you're feeling and act accordingly. If you feel dizzy, stop and rest. If the feeling persists, consult your doctor.

Ask for help if you need it. If someone is watching you move, they can also help correct your position for optimal results. And don't forget that you're getting stronger each time you practice these exercises. Give yourself a pat on the back for taking ownership of your body!

Exercising at the Right Level

It is very important as you're exercising to self-monitor how hard you are working. I am including two recommended ways to monitor yourself and determine if you are exercising at the right level, The Talk Test and The Rating of Perceived Exertion (RPE) scale.[14] Let's begin with the Talk Test. Think about speaking a sentence:

- If you can speak the whole sentence without stopping and are not feeling breathless, then you can exercise harder.
- If you cannot speak or can only say one word at a time and are severely breathless, then you are exercising too hard.
- If you can speak a sentence, take pauses to catch your breath, and are moderately breathless, then you are exercising at the right level.

Remember that it is normal to feel breathless when you exercise, and it is not harmful or dangerous. Gradually building your fitness can help you become less breathless. In order to improve your fitness, you should feel moderately breathless when you exercise.

The RPE is a scale used in the fitness world to subjectively measure how hard you're working during

---

[14] Productive Fitness, 2016.

exercise: that is, how much you're exerting yourself. Several scales are available, but I prefer the 1–10 RPE scale by Productive Fitness, which also includes the Talk Test. If you've ever spent time in a gym or fitness centre, you may have seen this poster on the wall—I know I have.

Here's a breakdown of the Exertion Scale, the corresponding zones, and their description of the Talk Test:

Exertion Scale	Zone	Talk Test
1/2	Inactive	Normal breathing; can talk normally
3/4	Health Improvement Zone	Light to moderate breathing; can carry on a conversation
5/6	Fitness Zone	Heavy breathing; only able to complete 1-2 sentences
7/8	Performance Zone	Heavier breathing; broken sentences or speaking only in syllables
9/10	High Performance Zone	Very heavy breathing; can't talk

A scale of 1 to 10 makes sense to most people, and it's something they can quickly comprehend. Level one represents low activity like standing—a minimal exertion with the ability to talk and breathe normally. Level 10 represents maximum intensity—a high performance zone with "severe" exertion and gasping for breath like you're trying to win a race. And, of course, every level from 1 to 10 represents an incremental increase in exertion that corresponds to a decrease in the ability to talk and breathe as you would while at rest. Makes sense, don't you think?

When I'm teaching classes or training people, I regularly reference the RPE scale because I believe that different activities should be performed at different levels. Unless you're an elite athlete or a weekend warrior in competition, is there really a need to perform at level 9/10? A rhetorical question, to which I would say, "No." And for the purposes of the exercises in this book, you want to focus on level 3/4—the "health improvement zone."

You will see this scale repeated in the exercise section of the book, so you don't need to continually flip back and forth.

How to Approach the Exercises

Finding time to do these exercises doesn't have to be complicated. When I work with clients in their homes, I send follow-up emails that list and describe the exercises we've done together. My goal is to make clients comfortable doing the exercises on their own.

In many cases, they write out the exercises on a sheet of paper for quick reference. You know, something that they can leave on the counter and refer to throughout the day. They often tell me that their list allows them to tackle the exercises one at a time, without feeling overwhelmed. This book is *your* quick reference guide. You can start with just one exercise, try them all in one session, or follow one of the workout plans—keep reading for more details. Whatever works for you. Regardless of how you approach them, you will benefit from incorporating these exercises into your daily life.

Most of the exercises are accompanied by one or two illustrations to get you started, as well as step-by-step instructions. At the end of the description, you'll find modifications on how to make an exercise easier or harder.

There are also two additional sections to help you with the exercises. The first includes a chart with each exercise listed and the goal(s) of the exercise, be it balance, posture, strength, and/or flexibility. You will see that many of these exercises achieve more than one goal.

The second section includes four sample workouts, based on the exercise goals you may want to achieve. For each of the goals listed in the previous section—balance, posture, strength, and flexibility—there is a gentle seated workout for you to follow.

Balance Definitions

Before you work through the exercises, let's revisit the basics of your balance system and the related definitions.

Our balance system is complex and relies on sensory input from three distinct systems: visual, vestibular, and proprioceptive (one component of the somatosensory system). All of this is just a fancy way of describing how our bodies process information. Let me break them down.

Visual system: This is about your eyes, which provide visual input to your brain as you move through life.

Vestibular system: This is the medical terminology for your inner ear, which processes sensory information about motion, equilibrium, and spatial orientation.

Proprioception (one component of the somatosensory system): This is your brain's ability to sense your body's position in space, via input from joints, muscles, and tendons.

NOTE: The Finger Follow exercise targets the visual and vestibular systems, while all of the exercises listed work the somatosensory system via proprioception.

What's the Speed Limit?

When you move on to the exercise section, you'll see that many of my instructions say things like, "slowly," or "with control." My intention is to have you focus on controlled movement that helps to strengthen the muscles being targeted, but also to prevent a fall. You're doing these exercises because you've identified a need for improvement in muscle strength. Sometimes, we may want to rush moves—if, for example, we find them difficult and want to complete them faster.

But executing the sequences too quickly is problematic for a few reasons. First, you won't necessarily strengthen the muscles correctly because you will be relying instead on momentum to move, not muscle power. Second, you're more likely to slouch in your chair (further impeding the good work of your muscles) if you're rushing.

If you're reading this book, I'm going to assume that your fitness goals are about enjoying your golden years without injuries sustained from falls. So, here's my advice to you as you tackle the exercises:

- Take it slow,
- Take breaks as needed,
- Remember that Rome wasn't built in a day and neither were you, and
- Focus on the goal of your exercise plan.

Please Keep Breathing

It's very important to remember to breathe as you complete the exercises. That's because holding your breath when you're exerting your body can place unnecessary strain on your heart. A helpful rule of thumb is to inhale and exhale for each step. For example: Inhale to complete step 1, exhale to complete step 2. Repeat. Depending on which part of an exercise sequence you find most difficult, you'll want to modify your breathing so that you're exhaling on the most strenuous portion. If you inhale during the most difficult part, you're more likely to hold your breath at the end of the inhalation.

Don't Forget to Warmup

If you're wondering about warmups, let's chat about that now. The purpose of a warmup is to prepare your body for the exercises you are about to do, that is, the workout you're preparing to undertake. A warmup gets your blood pumping, gradually and safely increasing your heart rate and blood circulation. It loosens up stiff joints and delivers blood to the muscles you're about to use, preventing the risk of an injury.

Even if you're planning to tackle these exercises one at a time—that is, one exercise per day—your body will still benefit from warming up for at least

two minutes. But don't worry, it doesn't have to be complicated. Here are three simple seated moves you can do to get warmed up and ready to exercise:
- One minute of seated marching,
- 30 seconds of shoulder rolls, and
- 30 seconds of arm swings.

If none of these appeal to you, turn on your favourite song and dance (seated or standing) for a few minutes. You might also use music to keep time as you complete the warmup suggestions I listed above.

Are you reading to begin? Then let's get started.

Chapter Three:
The Exercises

Rating of Perceived Exertion (RPE) Scale

Once again, here's the breakdown of the Exertion Scale, the corresponding zones, and their description of the Talk Test. For the purposes of this exercise guide, aim to be working in the Health Improvement Zone, also known as levels 3 to 4.

Exertion Scale	Zone	Talk Test
1/2	Inactive	Normal breathing; can talk normally
3/4	Health Improvement Zone	Light to moderate breathing; can carry on a conversation
5/6	Fitness Zone	Heavy breathing; only able to complete 1-2 sentences
7/8	Performance Zone	Heavier breathing; broken sentences or speaking only in syllables
9/10	High Performance Zone	Very heavy breathing; can't talk

Active Sitting

Exercise	Balance	Posture	Strength	Flexiblity
Active Sitting		x	x	

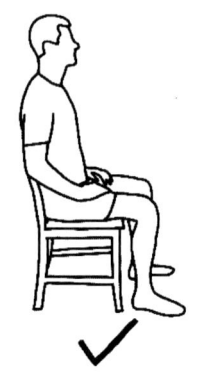

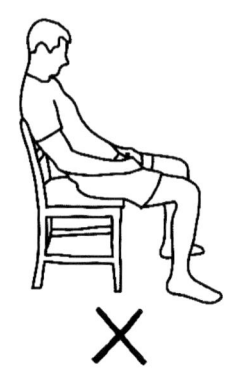

Active sitting helps us load our muscles and bones to fight the effects of gravity. Instead of outsourcing the role of our muscles by slumping in our seats, we should sit tall.

To start: Begin by sitting in a kitchen or dining room chair that has a firm seat.

1. Shifting forward: Slide your bottom forward so you're not leaning back in the chair. Place both feet flat on the floor in front of you. If your legs are shorter and you can't touch the floor, you can place a large book or block on the floor to support your feet. Don't roll onto your tailbone. Imagine you have a tail and you want the tail

behind you so you can wag it. Often, people roll backwards so they're resting on their tailbone instead of their sit bones — these are the bony part of your bum, the lower edge of your pelvis.
2. Shoulder position: Drop your shoulders away from your ears. It should feel like you're letting them slide down your back.
3. Head position: Pull your head and neck back so your ears are sitting over your shoulders, not pushed forward. Your head is now positioned over your centre of gravity, which is allowing you to strengthen your bones by loading them. Feel your muscles and bones at work.
4. Aim for five minutes of active sitting every hour.

Visualize: A string is tied to the top of your head, pulling you up towards the ceiling.

Do you need to make it easier? Start with two minutes of active sitting.

Are you ready to make it harder? Try for 10 minutes of active sitting every hour.

Seated Finger Follow

Exercise	Balance	Posture	Strength	Flexiblity
Seated Finger Follow	x		x	

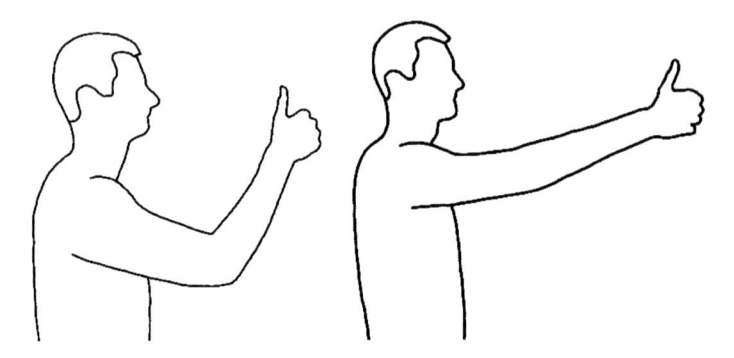

The Finger Follow is an eye-tracking exercise that helps improve balance by focusing on your visual and vestibular systems. Eye tracking exercises counteract deterioration that is a natural part of aging. The head movements will improve your ability to look around while your body is in motion throughout your day.

To start: Sit comfortably in a chair. A dining room chair with no arms is best for optimal movement.

Remember: If you feel dizzy during the exercise, stop and look straight ahead until the feeling passes.

1. Visual only: Using either hand, make a fist and stick your thumb towards the sky. Lift your hand in front of your face at eye level, approximately 12 inches away. Keep your arm bent at the elbow and hold your hand in this position.

2. Side to side: Slowly move your arm to the left, watching your thumb with both eyes, without moving your head or neck. This is a small movement because only your eyes are moving. Slowly move your arm back to the middle, and then to the right, and back to the middle again—always following with just your eyes.
3. Down and up: Continue tracking your thumb with both eyes as you slowly move your arm towards the floor, then back to the middle, up to the ceiling, and back to the middle again.
4. Visual and vestibular: Do Steps 1 to 3 a second time, but this time, stretch your arm straight out in front of you with no bend at the elbow. Follow your thumb with your eyes and your head as you move your arm through the same positions: left, middle, right, middle, down, middle, up, middle.

Do you need to make it easier? Take breaks between each movement.

Are you ready to make it harder? Repeat steps 1 to 4 a second time.

Seated Joint Mobility

Exercise	Balance	Posture	Strength	Flexiblity
Seated Joint Mobility	x			x

CARs—Controlled Articular Rotations—involve making s-l-o-w, controlled circles that increase mobility in your joints. Drawing these circles helps you feel less stiff and move more fluidly. Remember, motion is lotion! Some of these joint mobility exercises can be completed standing, seated, or lying down, and are thus repeated in the standing and lying down exercise sections. The key is to make slow and controlled movements. Many times, I see people drawing fast and sloppy circles. Fight the urge to get through the exercises as quickly as possible. Try to make the circular movements last for at least the number of seconds listed in the instructions.

Neck

To start: Sit comfortably in a chair. A dining room chair with no arms is best for optimal movement.

1. Clockwise: Looking straight ahead, rotate your head in a clockwise direction for five seconds.
2. Counterclockwise: Switch directions and repeat as you count another five seconds.

Visualize: The movement should look as if you're drawing a circle with the tip of your nose.

Do you need to make it easier? Count fewer seconds to complete the joint rotations, or repeat the sequence fewer times. Take breaks and rest.

Are you ready to make it harder? Please don't try to make it harder. CARs are a feel-good movement designed to keep your joints mobile. We don't want to force them to work harder, just better!

Shoulders

To start: Sit comfortably in a chair. A dining room chair with no arms is best for optimal movement.
1. Joint position: Relax your shoulders and keep your arms dropped at your side.
2. Forward: Slowly roll your shoulders forward, up, back, and down as you count to five.
3. Backward: Repeat in the opposite direction: pull them down, back, up, and forward as you count another five seconds.
4. Repeat: Repeat this sequence five to ten times.

Visualize: The movement should look as if your shoulders are a carpet that you are unrolling.

Do you need to make it easier? Count fewer seconds to complete the joint rotations, or repeat the sequence fewer times. Take breaks and rest.

Are you ready to make it harder? Please don't try to make it harder. CARs are a feel-good movement designed to keep your joints mobile. We don't want to force them to work harder, just better!

Elbows

To start: Sit comfortably in a chair. A dining room chair with no arms is best for optimal movement.

1. Joint position: Lift your arms out to the side at a slight angle. Bend your elbows so that your hands are pointing towards the floor.
2. Clockwise: Slowly make circles by rotating your lower arm—below the elbow—clockwise for five seconds.
3. Counterclockwise: Repeat in the other direction for another five seconds.
4. Repeat: Repeat this sequence five to ten times. Lower your arms to your sides when you are finished.

Visualize: Your arms look like a scarecrow and the rest of your body is a tin man, so the only joint able to move in this position is your elbow. Your fingers are slowly drawing circles on the ground.

Do you need to make it easier? Count fewer seconds to complete the joint rotations, or repeat the sequence fewer times. Take breaks and rest.

Are you ready to make it harder? Please don't try to make it harder. CARs are a feel-good movement designed to keep your joints mobile. We don't want to force them to work harder, just better!

Wrists

To start: Sit comfortably in a chair. A dining room chair with no arms is best for optimal movement.
1. Joint position: Lift your hands in front of you at chest height.
2. Clockwise: Slowly rotate both of your wrists in a clockwise direction while you count to ten.
3. Counterclockwise: Slowly rotate your wrists in the opposite direction while you count to ten again.
4. Repeat: Repeat this sequence five to ten times. Lower your hands to your sides when you are finished.

Visualize: Two pots of jam are being held in front of you and your hands are slowly stirring the thick spread.

Do you need to make it easier? Count fewer seconds to complete the joint rotations, or repeat the sequence fewer times. Take breaks and rest. Complete the movement as a lying down exercise.

Are you ready to make it harder? Please don't try to make it harder. CARs are a feel-good movement designed to keep your joints mobile. We don't want to force them to work harder, just better!

Fingers

To start: Sit comfortably in a chair. A dining room chair with no arms is best for optimal movement.

1. Joint position: Lift your hands in front of you and spread out your fingers. You will work both hands at the same time.
2. Clockwise: Starting with your pinky fingers, slowly draw circles with each pinky finger in a clockwise direction for five seconds.
3. Counterclockwise: Repeat in the opposite direction for five more seconds.
4. Repeat: Repeat circles in both directions with each finger. So after you have finished with your pinky fingers, move on to your ring fingers, then your middle fingers, and your index fingers. When it's time to work your thumbs, slow down the circles even more. They have a bigger range of motion, so try to make circles with them for seven to eight seconds in each direction.

Visualize: Two pots of jam are being held in front of you and your fingers are slowly stirring the thick spread.

Do you need to make it easier? Count fewer seconds to complete the joint rotations, or repeat the sequence fewer times. Take breaks and rest. Complete the movement as a lying down exercise.

Are you ready to make it harder? Please don't try to make it harder. CARs are a feel-good movement designed to keep your joints mobile. We don't want to force them to work harder, just better!

Waist

To start: Sit on the front edge of a chair with your feet planted on the ground. This will give you clearance to circle towards the back without hitting the back of your chair.

1. Clockwise: Slowly rotate your upper body in a clockwise circle as you count to five.
2. Counterclockwise: Repeat in a counterclockwise circle for five more seconds.
3. Repeat: Repeat this sequence five to ten times.

Visualize: You are a puppet, and the strings attached to your waist are being moved to slowly lean you forwards and then back, in a circular pattern.

Do you need to make it easier? Count fewer seconds to complete the joint rotations, or repeat the sequence fewer times. Take breaks and rest.

Are you ready to make it harder? Please don't try to make it harder. CARs are a feel-good movement designed to keep your joints mobile. We don't want to force them to work harder, just better!

Ankles

To start: Sit comfortably in a chair.
1. Joint position: Lift your right foot off the ground and bend your knee.
2. Clockwise: Count to ten as you draw circles with your foot by rotating your ankle in a clockwise direction.
3. Counterclockwise: Count to ten as you draw circles in the opposite direction.
4. Repeat: Repeat this sequence five to ten times, then lower your right foot to the ground.
5. Other ankle: Lift your left foot off the ground and repeat the entire sequence in both directions, then lower your left foot to the ground.
6. You can even try wiggling your toes a little. These aren't rotations, just an additional feel-good movement.

Visualize: Your foot is a pencil and you are using it to slowly draw circles on the ground.

Do you need to make it easier? Count fewer seconds to complete the joint rotations, or repeat the sequence fewer times. Take breaks and rest. Complete the movement as a lying down exercise.

Are you ready to make it harder? Please don't try to make it harder. CARs are a feel-good movement designed to keep your joints mobile. We don't want to force them to work harder, just better!

Seated Clock Toe Taps

Exercise	Balance	Posture	Strength	Flexiblity
Seated Clock Toe Taps				x

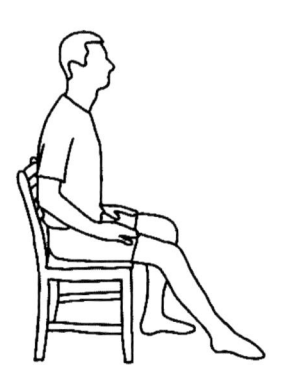

Clock toe taps as a seated exercise focus on hip mobility, as you straighten and bend your leg, rotating it in the hip socket.

To start: Sit on the edge of a sturdy chair. A dining room chair with no arms is best for optimal movement. Make sure there are no obstacles in a semi-circle in front of you.

1. Twelve o'clock: Reach your right foot forward with a straight leg and gently tap your big toe at the 12 o'clock position, then return it to the ground beside your left foot.
2. Moving around the clock: Continue tapping your toe around the imaginary clock, always returning to the centre between each

"hour" and placing your foot on the ground before continuing to the next "hour."
3. At the three o'clock position, repeat in the opposite direction, returning to 12 o'clock.
4. Switch legs: Repeat the toe taps with your left foot, beginning at 12 o'clock and working backwards from 11 o'clock down to nine o'clock. Repeat in the opposite direction, returning to 12 o'clock.
5. Try to do this exercise three times on each side.

Visualize: Imagine that there's a clock face on the floor and you're standing in the middle of it. The goal is to tap each hour on the clock from 12 o'clock all the way to six o'clock, and then repeat the toe taps in the opposite direction back to 12 o'clock.

Do you need to make it easier? If a particular position feels too difficult or uncomfortable, don't reach as far. Instead of tapping the toe on the ground, just lift the leg in that direction and return it to the centre, beside your other foot. Start by doing the exercises once on each leg, and gradually work your way up to three repetitions.

Are you ready to make it harder? Increase the number of repetitions to 5 to 8 on each side.

Double Gas Pedal

Exercise	Balance	Posture	Strength	Flexiblity
Double Gas Pedal	x		x	x

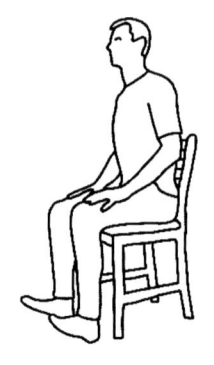

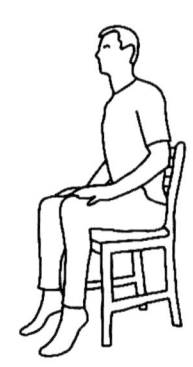

The gas pedal sequence will loosen up stiff ankles and strengthen the muscles in your calves and shins, thereby making walking easier and more fluid. Sitting at the front of the chair, rather than relying on the chair back for support, will further strengthen your core (aka your abdominal muscles). This exercise can be done wearing shoes or with bare feet.

To start: Sit tall in a chair, with both feet planted flat on the floor, hip-width apart. Look straight ahead and keep your body tall throughout the sequence.

1. Moving both feet at the same time, lift your toes off the floor.
2. Lower the toes to the starting position.
3. Lift both heels off the floor.
4. Lower the heels to the starting position.

Repeat steps 1 to 4 at least 8 to 10 times.

Visualize: Your feet are a seesaw, moving up and down in a controlled fashion.

Do you need to make it easier? Focus on one foot at a time, then switch to the other foot.

Are you ready to make it harder? Complete a second set of 8 to 10 repetitions.

Heel Slides

Exercise	Balance	Posture	Strength	Flexiblity
Heel Slides	x		x	

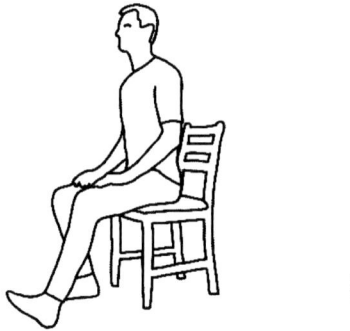

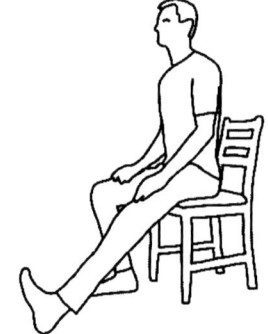

Heel slides work the muscles up the back of the leg, increasing lower limb strength and improving your walking stride. Sitting at the front of the chair, instead of relying on the chair back to hold your body upright, will further strengthen your core (aka your abdominal muscles). This exercise is best performed while wearing socks to allow your foot to move more freely.

To start: Sit tall in a chair, with both feet planted flat on the floor, hip-width apart. Look straight ahead and keep your body tall throughout the sequence.

1. Straighten your right leg and flex your right foot, so your heel remains in contact with the ground, but your toes are pointing up towards the ceiling.

2. Squeeze your bum muscles and the back of your thigh, using these muscle groups to drag your right heel back towards the chair while it remains in contact with the floor.
3. Reverse the movement and slide your heel away from you, straightening your right knee until you reach the starting position.
4. Perform 10–12 repetitions on the right side.
5. Repeat steps 1 to 4 with the left foot.

Visualize: Imagine driving a car with no hand break and you are on a hill, slide the leg out to push down on the brake pedal (squeeze your bum muscles to hold it there). Then, release the brake slowly as you slide your heel back towards the chair.

Do you need to make it easier? Stay closer to the chair (don't straighten your leg completely).

Are you ready to make it harder? Slide both heels out and back at the same time.

Torso Twists

Exercise	Balance	Posture	Strength	Flexiblity
Torso Twists		x	x	x

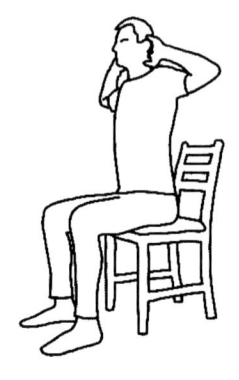

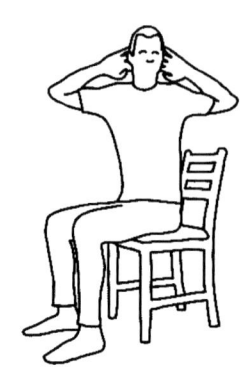

Torso twists work the abdominal muscles on the sides of your body, strengthening your core and improving the mobility of your spine. Both of these are important for maintaining good balance during functional activities, like twisting and turning as you empty your dishwasher or getting out of your car.

To start: Sit tall on a chair with your feet flat on the ground about hip-width apart. Make sure you don't lean back in the chair. Place your hands lightly behind your head, with your elbows bent and pointing out towards the sides of the room.

1. Slowly rotate your torso to the left as far as you comfortably can, keeping the rest of your body still, i.e. your bum doesn't move on the chair.

2. Rotate back to the starting position in the middle.
3. Continue rotating to the right side as far as you comfortably can, keeping the rest of your body still.
4. Rotate back to the starting position in the middle.
5. Repeat steps 1 to 4 at least eight to 10 times.

Visualize: Your body from your hips up to the top of your head is a key, turning as a solid unit back and forth in a lock.

Do you need to make it easier? Cross your arms in front of your chest to complete the sequence with a lower centre of gravity.

Are you ready to make it harder? Close your eyes to perform the torso twists, increasing the response of your vestibular and somatosensory systems.

Reverse Sit-ups

Exercise	Balance	Posture	Strength	Flexiblity
Reverse Situps	x	x	x	

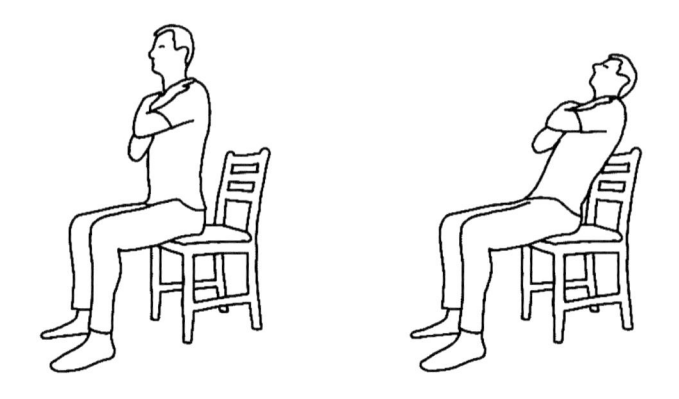

While everyone loves to hate sit-ups and other abdominal exercises, that's because they're targeting a part of our bodies that we often neglect. In addition to improving our core strength, sit-ups allow us to have better balance and stability, improved posture. They also reduce the risk of back pain and injury.

To start: Sit tall on the edge of a chair with both feet planted flat on the floor, hip-width apart. Look straight ahead and cross your arms over your chest, with each hand touching the opposite shoulder.

1. Slowly lean back, moving your torso as a solid unit towards the back of your chair. Stop before your shoulder blades touch the chair.

2. Pull your body forward in a smooth motion, returning yourself to the upright starting position.
3. Repeat steps 1 and 2 at least eight to 10 times.

Tighten your stomach as if you're about to be tickled by your grandchild. Maintain that level of stiffness throughout the sequence.

Do you need to make it easier? Hook your hands on the sides of the chair, and follow steps 1 and 2.

Are you ready to make it harder? Bring your hands up beside your head, palms facing forward, elbows bent, with your fingertips touching your temples. Keep your hands in this position and follow steps 1 and 2.

Side to Side Arm Reaches

Exercise	Balance	Posture	Strength	Flexiblity
Side to Side Arm Reaches	x	x	x	

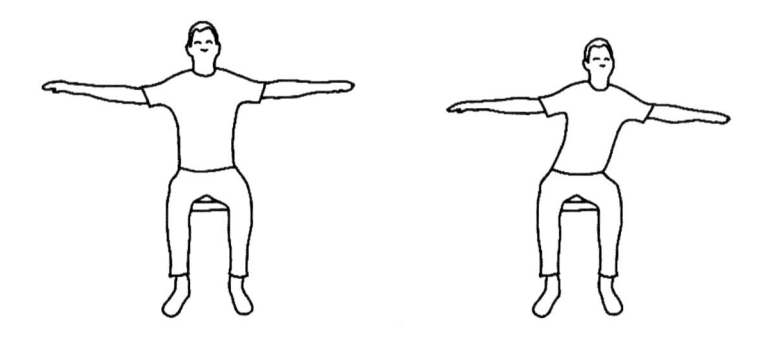

Side-to-side arm reaches work the abdominal muscles on the sides of your body, strengthening your core and improving the mobility of your spine.

To start: Sit tall on the edge of a chair, with both feet planted flat on the floor, hip-width apart. Look straight ahead. Lift your arms out to the side at shoulder height, with your elbows straightened.

1. Keeping your bum and hips planted on the chair, slowly lean your torso towards your left side, as if you're trying to touch something at shoulder height with your left hand. Don't tip your hand towards the floor.
2. Return to the centre, with your torso forming a straight line towards the ceiling.

3. Repeat the movement towards your right side.
4. Return to the centre starting position.
5. Follow steps 1 to 4 at least eight to 10 times.

Visualize: Your torso is bound by a metal cage, and your arms are the ropes in an evenly-matched tug of war.

Do you need to make it easier? Hook your hands on the sides of the chair, and follow steps 1 to 4.

Are you ready to make it harder? Follow steps 1 to 4, reaching even farther out to each side.

Seated Overhead Arm Raises

Exercise	Balance	Posture	Strength	Flexiblity
Seated Overhead Arm Raises		x	x	

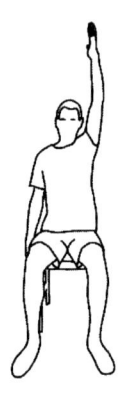

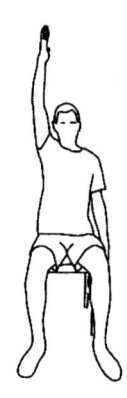

Our torso can help keep us upright for exercises like overhead arm reaches. This improves our posture, strengthening both our muscles and our bones. When we stand straighter, it is easier to walk with a straighter frame and see where we are going, thus reducing the likelihood of a momentum-based fall. These reaches will help you achieve that goal and keep you from toppling forward when you're walking.

To start: Sit comfortably in a chair. A dining room chair with no arms is best for optimal movement.

1. Lift your right arm above your head, straightening the elbow and maintaining a tall posture.

2. Lower your right arm to the starting position.
3. Lift your left arm above your head, straightening the elbow and maintaining a tall posture.
4. Lower your left arm to the starting position.
5. Continue alternating arm reaches until you have completed 10 on each side.

Visualize: You are a puppet, and the string holding up your head and torso is taut and unmoving, while the strings on your wrists alternately lift your arms upwards.

Do you need to make it easier? Focus on lifting your arm as high as possible, keep the elbow bent as needed.

Are you ready to make it harder? Complete another set of 10, alternating sides each time.

Seated Wall Push-up

Exercise	Balance	Posture	Strength	Flexiblity
Seated Wall Pushup		x	x	

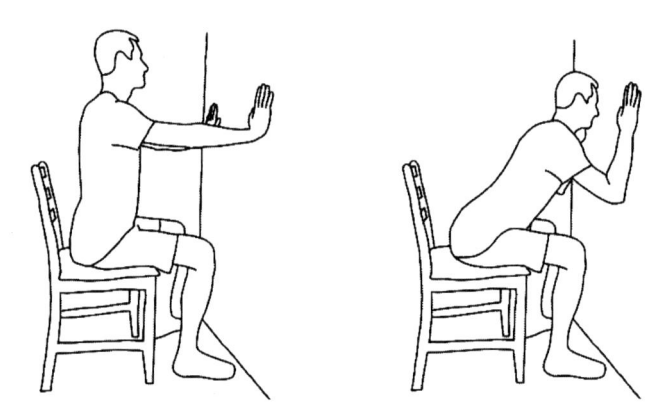

Push-ups are an effective exercise to build upper body strength. Your chest, shoulders, back, and arms all work together to move you with control. Your abdominal muscles also play a role in maintaining a stiff torso and preventing you from arching your back, thereby strengthening your entire core.

To start: Sit on a chair with your feet flat on the ground and your bum close to the edge of the chair. The chair should be close enough to the door/wall that when you lean forward, you won't fall off the chair.

1. Place your open palms against the door/wall, directly in front of your shoulders. Relax your shoulders down away

from your ears, and squeeze your stomach muscles.
2. Check your elbows, they should be almost straight (not locked) in the starting position.
3. Slowly bend your elbows to bring your nose closer to the wall or door.
4. Straighten your arms to return to the starting position.
5. Repeat steps 3 and 4 at least five to 10 times.

Visualize: Your body from your shoulders down to your hips is a solid board, that moves as a single unit.

Do you need to make it easier? Don't lower yourself as close to the door/wall, keep a bigger bend in your elbows.

Are you ready to make it harder? Do a second set of 5 to 10 repetitions.

Seated Side Bends

Exercise	Balance	Posture	Strength	Flexiblity
Seated Side Bends		x	x	

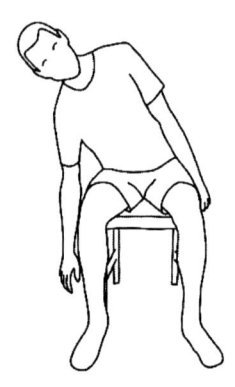

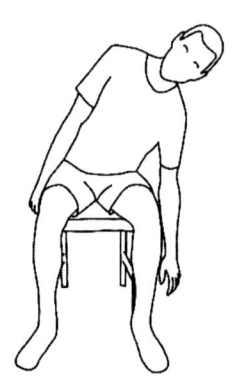

Side bends work the muscles along the sides of your torso, helping to increase your upper body strength and maintain an upright posture.

To start: Sit comfortably in a chair. A dining room chair with no arms is best for optimal movement.

1. Place your arms at your sides, fingertips facing down towards the floor.
2. At your waist, lean to your right side with your fingertips reaching towards the floor.
3. Move back to your starting position.
4. Continue bending to the right and up again five to 10 times.
5. Follow steps 1 to 4 on the left side.

Visualize: You're a teapot wedged between two sheets of glass, tipping over from the waist without leaning forward or back.

Do you need to make it easier? Start with 3 to 5 repetitions. Take frequent breaks and rest.

Are you ready to make it harder? Increase the number of repetitions to 8 to 10.

Seated Knee Straightener

Exercise	Balance	Posture	Strength	Flexiblity
Seated Knee Straightener			x	x

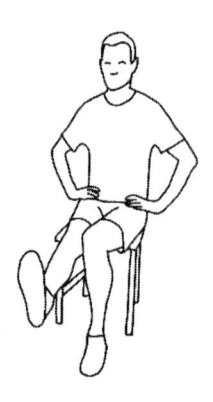

This exercise will help strengthen your leg muscles, boost your confidence, and improve your balance, thereby facilitating better movement when you're walking or moving throughout the day. Sitting at the front of the chair, rather than relying on the chair back for support, will further strengthen your core (aka your abdominal muscles). This exercise can be done wearing shoes or with bare feet.

To start: Sit tall in a chair, with both feet planted flat on the floor, hip-width apart. Look straight ahead and keep your body tall throughout the sequence.

1. Straighten one knee and hold your out straight for a moment.
2. Slowly lower your leg to the floor

3. Repeat steps 1 and 2 up to 10 times on the same leg.
4. Relax your first leg and repeat steps 1 to 3 on your other leg.

Visualize: Imagine you are trying to kick a ball straight up to the ceiling.

Do you want to make it easier? Do fewer repeats on each leg, aim for 3 to 5 times per leg to start.

Are you ready to progress? Increase the time holding your leg out straight to a count of 3 seconds. Perform the exercise more slowly.

Seated High March

Exercise	Balance	Posture	Strength	Flexiblity
Seated High March			x	

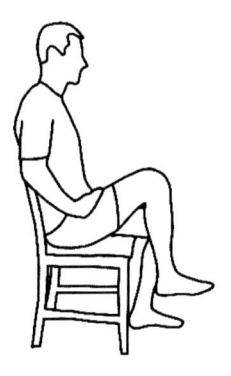

The seated high march is a strength exercise that creates stability on both sides of the body. You are working on your core stability, which helps with balance. Strong muscles and bones allow us to lift our legs and feet over obstacles, and avoid shuffling when walking, which can lead to falls.

To start: Sit on a chair with your feet flat on the ground and your bum close to the edge of the chair. Try to sit as tall as you can.

1. Lift: Lift one knee up as high as you can and hold it up for three to five seconds.
2. Lower: Use control to lower the leg to the starting position. (Don't use gravity!)
3. Repeat: Repeat Steps 1 and 2 on the other leg.

4. Aim for ten marches, alternating sides with each repetition.

Visualize: Your torso, from just above your hips right up to the top of your head, is frozen in a solid block of ice, and you can only move your legs up and down.

Do you need to make it easier? Start with as many as you can, and work your way up to ten. Take a break between each repetition.

Are you ready to make it harder? Do a second set of 10 marches.

Appendix:
Exercise Breakdown, Sample Workouts, & Activity Logs

The exercises in this book will help you strengthen your body, enhance your posture, increase your balance and coordination, and improve your energy—all of which work together to reduce your risk of falling. The chart below highlights which exercises accomplish which goals. So, for example, if you only have a few minutes and want to work on your posture, you can easily see which one or two exercises you might want to complete. And the workout plans on the next page show you how to put a workout together based on specific goals.

Exercise	Balance	Posture	Strength	Flexiblity
Active Sitting		x	x	
Seated Finger Follow	x		x	
Seated Joint Mobility	x			x
Seated Clock Toe Taps				x
Double Gas Pedal	x		x	x
Heel Slides	x		x	
Torso Twists		x	x	x
Reverse Situps	x	x	x	
Side to Side Arm Reaches	x	x	x	
Seated Overhead Arm Raises		x	x	
Seated Wall Pushup		x	x	
Seated Side Bends		x	x	
Seated Knee Straightener			x	x
Seated High March			x	

Below, you will find four sample workouts to help you focus on specific exercise goals.

1. **Balance**
   - Seated Finger Follow, p. 42
   - Heel Slides, p. 58
   - Seated Side to Side Arm Reaches, p. 64
   - Reverse Sit-Up, p. 62
   - Double Gas Pedal, p. 56

2. **Posture**
   - Active Sitting, p. 40
   - Torso Twists, p. 60
   - Seated Wall Push-up, p. 68
   - Seated Overhead Arm Raises, p. 66
   - Seated Side Bends, p. 70

3. **Strength**
   - Seated Wall Push-up, p. 68
   - Seated Side Bends, p. 70
   - Seated High March, p. 74
   - Seated Knee Straightener, p. 72
   - Seated Overhead Arm Raises, p. 66

4. **Flexibility**
   - Seated Joint Mobility: neck, shoulders, elbows, wrist, fingers, waist, ankles, pp. 45–52
   - Seated Clock Toe Taps, p. 54
   - Double Gas Pedal, p. 56

Checking In With Yourself

The following pages contains one week's worth of daily logs to track how you're feeling and the hard work you've completed. Some days, you may not feel up to completing your exercises. That's okay. If you do feel up to recording your progress, I hope you'll see that you're on the right path. Every minute of movement counts, and gentle exercise will help you feel better and reduce your risk of falling. Exercise can improve your sense of control, coping ability, and self-esteem.

Your daily living activities, such as housecleaning, food preparation, grocery shopping, and gardening, are considered light physical activity. If you want to record these activities in the exercise category, go for it. It counts, and seeing it written down may help you feel better about what may sometimes seem to you like little progress.

	Day: _____
How are you feeling, really? Physically and mentally	
What exercises did you do? Remember, "none" is also a valid response.	
What did you do today that made you feel good?	
Did you drink enough water today?	

	Day: _____
How are you feeling, really? Physically and mentally	
What exercises did you do? Remember, "none" is also a valid response.	
What did you do today that made you feel good?	
Did you drink enough water today?	

	Day: _____
How are you feeling, really? Physically and mentally	
What exercises did you do? Remember, "none" is also a valid response.	
What did you do today that made you feel good?	
Did you drink enough water today?	

	Day: _____
How are you feeling, really? Physically and mentally	
What exercises did you do? Remember, "none" is also a valid response.	
What did you do today that made you feel good?	
Did you drink enough water today?	

	Day: _____
How are you feeling, really? Physically and mentally	
What exercises did you do? Remember, "none" is also a valid response.	
What did you do today that made you feel good?	
Did you drink enough water today?	

	Day: _____
How are you feeling, really? Physically and mentally	
What exercises did you do? Remember, "none" is also a valid response.	
What did you do today that made you feel good?	
Did you drink enough water today?	

	Day: _____
How are you feeling, really? Physically and mentally	
What exercises did you do? Remember, "none" is also a valid response.	
What did you do today that made you feel good?	
Did you drink enough water today?	

Reviews and Testimonials

"I carry *Balance and Your Body* in my bag, between my cell phone and wallet, so I always have it nearby as reference. The exercises are basic and you can easily incorporate them in our daily life, and if you don't remember them, you can do what I do."

— Monique

"This was fabulous! Thanks so much for providing this."

— How Can Seniors Prevent a Fall workshop participant

"I really enjoyed *Balance and Your Body*! I had fun doing the exercises with my parents (aged 88 and 87). It gets them going, as well as me. It all makes sense—you have to read it and start exercising."

—Teresa

"*Balance and Your Body* is Amanda's second book especially written for seniors. The message is simple and true: "Move more, stay healthy longer!" The book is well organized and fun to read; the exercises are easy to follow and can be practiced whenever you have some time throughout the day (or sleepless night). No gym or equipment required!"

—An enthusiastic senior

"Her new book, *Balance and Your Body*, is very clear and easy to read. She explains why we need to move and the different aspects of balance. The exercises are simple and drawings help understand them. Not at all overwhelming to do the exercises. A very helpful book for any senior concerned about maintaining their independence. Essential for seniors to stay independent. Well done!"

—Amazon customer

"A well researched and written handbook. Just what's needed for anyone requiring the ability to improve their balance most likely senior citizens."

— Amazon customer, *Balance and Your Body*

"I use the exercises daily."

— Amazon customer, *Balance 2.0*

About the Author

Amanda Sterczyk is an independent author and personal trainer based in Ottawa, Canada. In 2016, she founded The Move More Institute™, an initiative to promote healthy active living and teach individuals how to sneak "exercise" into their daily lives. Her slogan is "Move more, feel better." Amanda holds a Master's degree in social psychology from Carleton University. *Chair Exercises for Fall Prevention* is her tenth book.

You can connect with Amanda online by visiting her website: www.amandasterczyk.com.

Made in United States
Cleveland, OH
24 March 2025